Table of Contents

....

<u>PROLOGUE</u>

Shooting pain in body joints and afflictions in muscles create appalling state for a mortal. The causes could be negligence about health or lazy life style with sheer ease...

To topple with this nuisance unease... "Savants"... World fame holder, give exemplary services to drop off the joints pain and muscles afflictions and their remedies are recognized for hundreds of years.

Within the facts.. ...... A panel of investigators completed review for more than 500 controlled trials to look at the patients, using any cure from the "Savants" and in the book. Crosswise, Panel studies, their assessment confirmed nearly zero side effect on the health of all these remedies..... In addition, Panel studies are placed side by side, these most accepted Cures for years by "Savants" not appropriate only for Joints pain and Muscles Afflictions but also appreciably decrease the hazard of numerous deceases carefully. If anyone apprehensive by Joints pain and Muscles Afflictions and anxious to get rid of, then these Cures will definitely with a sheer thorough guarantee without a bit of uncertainty, will cure with 100% recovery.

"IN FACT, SHOCKING TRUTH WITH ENTIRE RECUPERATION WILL START REPAIRING FROM THE DAY ONE"

How I cross this extremely vast, full with clutters passage and depart in this arena to collect the Composed Cures from the disciples of the world fame holders "SAVANTS" for the mankind benevolence those are tired of the unlike ways of treatments and medicinal drugs. This is a long journey full of hurdles and obstacles. I fight hard for the Composed Cures.

To patients and every suffering person of Joints pain and Muscles Afflictions, bearing pain, pressure... For wiping up the turmoil of joints pain and muscles afflictions with Composed Cures... Kindly focus on the CURES with imperative notes and hand over a blissful time. It's obvious that the given precedents are for all, those suffering by joints pain and muscles afflictions and eager or keen for a pain free life... I must request to all of them, please do not waste time more in vast study of pain free life and stick to any Cure from the book to definitively end result for the correction and repairing of ailment with100% convalescence.

Dr. Mohammad Anees

....

SYNOPSIS

Since the arrival of this entity (As
human being) on this planet, different
infectious deceases are also chasing
him and different individual, groups,
organization, companies are also
working to topple these different
infectious or contagious deceases.
Beside excellent, exceptional efforts in
the field of Joints pain and Muscles
Afflictions by the group of "Savant"....
All the Cures had influenced the keen
and anxious suffering persons with vast
satisfactions. Each cure enhances the
rapidity of muscle and correct the
joints moment with acceleration.

Certainly... This is not a outset or
inception of Cures for joint pains and
muscles afflictions, but when other
each attempt, the result is in a tragedy
and eventually patients are in the
avalanche of the glooms of despairs by
other way of treatments and
medications... Then Composed
Cures   lift the barriers down between
them, support and treat without any

5

side force to eliminate the deep joints pains and muscles afflictions. Patents retrieve and recover from this hurting epidemic pain ailment. Without suspicion, each choir will establish complimentary... Physically and emotionally to the patients without contradictions to enhance her/his desires for substantial joy with free painful life.

Author may request to pay heed to this rendition as a courtesy.......... One man supplicate after his prayer every day of his Almighty God, please bless me with Son.

Afterwards 10 years one Angle came from the sky and castigate him, you are repeating your request and supplicating after your prayer every day since ten years today. You marry first than supplicate for a son? Almighty God is with the supplication of his humanity? Narration is forwarded to the suffering persons (Patients)... If you are tired of others way of treatments and medications than avail this golden opportunity and follow any cure in Composed Cures for joint pains and muscles afflictions for your healthy life.

God bless all and pass through all the sweetness and healthy pain free life.

Dr. Mohammad Anees

....

About Author Mission

Before starting Composed Cures for joints pain and muscles afflictions. Kindly note, Author mission is straightforward, want to provide, those were tired by the different manner of treatments and medications already... Take advantage of this golden chance and enjoy joints pain and muscles afflictions, free life using any cure in this book for 100% recovery. Lifetime is around you and only once.... Take care about your health without wasting time.

"COMPOSED CURES ARE ULTIMATE RESTORE TO HEALTH FOR JOINTS PAIN AND MUSCLES AFFLICTIONS............ IF DIRECTLY FOLLOW TO ADMINISTRATE THE CURES"

Even though a great stack, in clumps and in bundles is written on pain subject, like......... There is but one perfect child in the world and every mother find in it. And If seeking authentic and real certain fact for perennial joints pain and muscles afflictions Cures than shocking truth in the name of Composed Cures is available.

....

Attention:

Thoughtfully pay concentration to below Imperative Notes.

Note.1

For Massage Time duration

Period of massage, for every Cure is, one month and duration is one hour.

Hopefully symptoms of joints pain and muscles afflictions will die altogether in a single month.

Get down to rub down every night before sleeping and one hour after breakfast in the morning without negligence. All the marijuana cigarettes and body parts must be cleaned with Luke warm water and dried with towel thoroughly before massage and must be handled with heavy ring, cloth or with a small blanket after the massage.

Note.2

BEFORE BREAKFAST IT'S ESSENTIAL.... Before taking routine breakfast with brown sugar and coffee (optional fried one egg, if asked). Hold handle of one tablespoonful Cinnamon in powder form 20 g, and two tablespoonfuls Acacia Honey 50 g, Keep cinnamon in powder form and Pure Honey from Acacia Tree by Small Bee, keep in stock for daily use in a kitchen shop.

Total Cinnamon in powder form needed 600 g, Acacia Honey 1.5 KG for 30 days.......

N.B.... Please pay attention that the patient is not suffering from diabetes and Pure Acacia small bee jungle Honey is used for Cures.....

If a patient is suffering from diabetic than kindly check the quality of Acacia Honey before using it? That it's really by Small Bee from Acacia tree or not? If doubt remains than use pure olive oil, one tablespoonful and ½ tablespoonful that honey and combine it with Cinnamon powder and follow the above instructions before getting breakfast. For breakfast follow Note 3.

Note.3

Take musk 2 g

Take saffron 2g

Hot water 2 cup

If you are a patient of diabetic, and then select your breakfast with brown bread slices and black chocolate with cream....... In addition maximum one fried egg and drink two cups hot water mixed with musk 2 g and saffron 2 g. Dissolve saffron leaves in low water and grind by hand with a small spoon

11

in the cup, until all the leaves are crushed and water become colored.

....

CURE NO.1

Get 1 (one) beetle leaf.... Masses used to masticate beetle leaf with other relish condiments in South East Asia...... Put one beetle leaf in a trough, fill with clean water under the sky in the eve. The area must be constructed of stiff mud and without any color (better)......

Take 1 g, Musk. 50 g, Royal Jelly.

In the morning, Take this drink before taking anything. Put one tablespoon full Royal Jelly and 1 (single) g Musk inside the drink before engaging in anything. Put water again to repeat the operation and change the beetle leaf when odor is changed or after every three days. Continue till symptom of joints pain and muscles afflictions reduced gradually and completely broke.

Total Beetle Leafs needed 20 pieces, Musk 60 g, Royal Jelly 3 KG for 30 days........

Take Trout Fish from River water 1 KG, or as needed by the patient for lunch and dinner, remove skin and thorn, head of Trout Fish and keep it aside separately. Cook Trout Fish in sunflower oil with garlic 50 g, Black Pepper, 50 g, Fresh ginger 50 g, Black seed 50 g, with salt to taste... Eat with brown bread or brown rice at lunch and dinner.

This is for one day, but patient responsible can stock all the supply (Trout fish and other constituents) in kitchen store from the market for 30 days or on a daily basis...

Put thorns, skin and head of Trout Fish in separate 200 g, sunflower oil and incinerate it. After straining it and create it in powder form. Put it in a bit of cloth and make like a small cushion and set along the joints where pain is pervasive. Smashed it with a bandage from further falling or moving from the point. Get rid of the cushion before massage every time and invest it again after massage every time.

Take Sesame oil 0.5 liter, Olive Oil 0.5 liter, Pumpkin seeds oil 0.5 liter and mix all vigorously than put in the pan. Take any River Fish Eggs 500 g, Tymol seeds 250 g, and cloves 250 g, in the oil and set the pan on fire. Cut all the factors and then sift it and put the oil in the bottle or a stadium. Clean all the marijuana cigarettes and body functions before applying oil and have it penetrate for 10 minutes then start massaging vigorously. After hacking through the marijuana cigarettes and body parts with cotton.

••

CURE NO. 2

Take 1 Jungle pigeon and slaughter it. Maintain all the blood of Jungle Pigeon in separate bowl. Apply blood to the joints and afflicted muscle body parts before lunch in the morning... let it dry and give it until cleaning prior to massage at night before sleeping as described under...

This is for one day need and for complete course of 30 days needs 30 pigeons.

 Get 1 (one) Jungle Pigeon or as needed by the patient for lunch and dinner. Cook in garlic 50 g, Black Pepper, 50 g, (BBQ) with salt to taste, Eat with brown sugar or brown rice at lunch and dinner.

This is for one day need, but patient responsible can stock all the supply (Pigeon and other parts) in kitchen store from the market for 30 days or on a daily basis.

Hold handle of one teaspoonful Aniseed (Fennel) in powder form and one teaspoonful pure olive oil with one tablespoonful Acacia Honey before sleeping after massage and repeat this process until symptoms died completely.

Take Walnut oil 250 g, Pumpkin seed oil, 500 g, Olive oil 500 g, Clove oil 250 g, mix all the oils and lay in the pan on fire. Take 12 jungle pigeon eggs. Burn all the eggs and then sift it and put the oil in the bottle or a stadium. Clean all the marijuana cigarettes and body sections were applied blood already............. Apply oil and have it penetrate for 10 minutes, then start massaging vigorously. After hacking through the marijuana cigarettes and body parts with cotton.

···

CURE NO. 3

Take 100 g, Black Chick Peas and soak in water in the evening after cleaning thoroughly. In the morning, drink all this water one hour after taking routine breakfast with brown bread, Acacia Honey and dark chocolate. And before breakfast, do not forget to catch a hold of one tablespoonful cinnamon in powder form and two tablespoons full Acacia

Honey before taking anything in the dawning...

Immediately take 1 KG Turkey meat, (or as needed by the patient) Take pumpkin seeds 100 g, Melon seeds 100 g, Raisin 200 g, Cashew nuts 200 g, (Roasted)

Take garlic 100 g, Black seed 100 g, Fresh ginger 200 g, Black pepper 100 g (Whole), Black cardamom 20 g... cooks all above in sunflower cooking oil in the way you like with salt to taste and eat with brown bread or brown rice at lunch and dinner.

This is for one day, but patient responsible can stock all the supply (Turkey meat and other voices) in kitchen store from the market for 30 days or on a daily basis.

Take Sesame oil 750 g, Olive oil 750 g and mix both oils. After mixing both oils, put the pan on fire.

Take Nutmeg 100 g, and crush it in grain size

Take 10 green shafts of Eggplants / Aubergine / Garden Egg. Vegetable Incinerate all above in the above mixed oil and after carefully sift it and place it in a separate bowl or in bottle for message.

While applying oil on joints for massage and on affected areas of body parts for muscles afflictions. Make slowly tapping with hands on joints and afflicted muscle areas to penetrate oil and leave for 15 transactions. After start massage on joints and afflicted muscle areas on whole body. Clean all the marijuana cigarettes and body parts before new message every day and embrace all the joints and body regions with heavy cotton.

....

CURE NO. 4

Take 2 KG long red dates, and require the seed away.

Take pine nut 200 g, with rind (without stripping down)...... After cleaning thoroughly all the pine nuts, toasted in olive oil....... Being away all the toasted pine nuts and squeezed it in grain size and mix with dates. Take Flaxseed 500 g, and toast with olive oil and mash it in powder form. Mix all the ingredients and Make equal weight of 60 balls or candy. Get hold of pure rose water as needed or Two liter (keep it for next exercise).... Eat one candy or ball before massage in the lunch and in the evening with pure rose water.

This is for one whole month to complete course of 30 days.

Now take venison meat 1 KG. (If available) otherwise take Eel Fish or any from river water. Place garlic and ginger paste thoroughly on venison meat or Eel Fish and make it BBQ for lunch and dinner. Eat with garlic and tomato sauce with brown bread or brown rice.

This is for one day, but patient responsible can stock all the supply (Venison meat or Eel Fish and other constituents) in kitchen store from the market for 30 days or on a daily basis........

Take hold of pure Rose petal Oil 1000 g, and olive oil 500 g, Mix both oils vigorously.

Clean all the areas of the physical structure and joints with Luke warm water and dry it completely.. (Pain full joints and afflicted muscle areas) after cleaning the joints and body, apply oil And leave for 10 transactions. Later taking up massage with firm hands and hand over the sticks and other parts of the body with heavy cotton.

....

CURE NO. 5

Take fresh Turmeric Vegetable 1 KG (its form is like fresh ginger)...... Take

1 KG Yellow or Pumpkin Trout Fish Eggs.

Pack 4 Black Cardamom, Black Pepper, 100 g, and garlic 200 g, make paste with fish   eggs and mix with Turmeric Veg. Cook in tomato sauce with sunflower cooking oil. Eat with brown bread or with brown rice in lunch and dinner.

This is for one day, but patient responsible can stock all the supply (Turmeric Veg. And other ingredients) in kitchen store from the market for 30 days or on a daily basis...

Now hold the two slices of melon... Eat melons with family and dry the rinds of the melons under the sunlight. After completely dried out crushed the dried rinds in grain size.

Get 6 fresh corn plant (Maize with Cases) with the rind and hares... Eat the corn and keep the rinds (cases) with hairs aside.

Take carrot bottom (green) 500 g, and put under the sun for dried up.

After completely dried out under the Sun, crush dried carrot bottom in grain size.

Now take five liter water in the can and put crushed carrot bottom, Corn plant crushed cases and hairs, Crushed Melon rinds inside and boil it until water remain half. Take one glass from this extract and put one tablespoonful Acacia Honey in and drink it in the afternoon, two hours before sunset. eep other material for adjacent use in refrigerator without sifts. Repeat till symptoms last forever or pain intensity and hurt getting reduced.

This is for 7 days (one week) but patient responsible can stock all the supply (Carrot bottom, Melon rinds, Corn plants rinds and hairs) in kitchen store for the securities industry for 30 days........

Take sesame oil 750 g, olive oil 750 g......... Mix both oil vigorously.

Take Mace 300 g, Tymol seeds 250 g, Dry ginger 250 g, Cumin seeds 250 g............ Mix both oils and put in the pan with all the elements in it. Place pan on the fire and incinerate all the ingredients. Tense up the oil and put in the bottle or a stadium.

Immediately clean all the joints and afflicted muscle areas body parts before massage with warm water and dry completely with a towel. Apply thin layer of oil and depart for 10 minutes to soak up. Get down to rub down with hard human beings. Cut through the sticks and other body parts after the massage. Continue massage as explained, till symptoms died forever.

....

CURE NO. 6

Take aniseed (Fennel) 10 g, Dry ginger10g, Cumin seed 10 g, Black seed 10 g. Put all the ingredients in the pan and toast it without oil and grind it in powder form and keep in safe bottle. Take one hour after your routine breakfast...... one tablespoon full powder of the above ingredients and swallow with 0.5 liter pure rose water and hold in dark red molasses 20 g, over this immediately.

This is for one day need and for complete course of 30 days needs accordingly.

Take Trout Fish 1 KG or as required by the patient... remove the skin and irritants and keep it separate aside. Take hold of dry fenugreek 100 g, Garlic 200 g, Dry Ginger 200 g, Black Pepper 100 g, Cloves 50 g...

Prepare pastes in 200 g corn flour and apply all the paste on Trout Fish. Make Trout Fish **BBQ** as you like and eat it with garlic sauce with brown bread or brown rice.

This is for one day, but patient responsible can stock all the supply (Trout Fish and other constituents) in kitchen store from the market for 30 days or on a daily basis...

Take Sesame oil 0.5 liter, Olive oil 0.5 liter, Pumpkin seeds oil 0.5 liter and mix all then put in the pan. Take Trout Fish river water fish, Eggs 500 g, Tymol (Common Hindi Name) seeds 250 g, Cloves 250 g, Mace 250 g, Skin and thorns of Trout fish already kept separate aside... Crush all before adding in oil and pan on fire. Cut all the factors and then strain the oil. Put the oil in the bottle or a stadium. Clean all the marijuana cigarettes and body functions before applying oil and have it penetrate for 10 minutes then start massaging vigorously. After hacking through the marijuana cigarettes and body parts with cotton.

....

CURE NO. 7

Take 4 Peahen eggs (If not available) than take 12 partridges eggs. Take 1.5 KG or 1.5 Liter sesame oil.

Take Mace 200 g, Nutmeg, 200 g, Black seed 200 g...

Invest all the eggs, ingredients, oil in the pan on fire and incinerate all the eggs, ingredients..... Strain the oil and keep in a bottle or bowl for massage on pain full joints and afflicted muscle areas on different body sections.

This is for complete one month for a massage. Hopefully symptoms of joints pain and muscles afflictions will die altogether....

Transfer the lamb meat from the neck, without white fat layer (all important)

Take hold of dry fenugreek 200 g, Garlic 200 g, Dry Ginger 200 g, Black Pepper 100 g, Cloves 50 g.......

Clean the meat and put all ingredients in the pan with 1.5 liter fresh water and boil the   mixture till water reduced 50% than drink this soup and eat meat/other ingredients with brown rice or brown bread at lunch and dinner.

This is for one day, but patient responsible can stock all the supply (lamb meat and other   parts) in kitchen store from the market for 30 days or on a daily basis...

Immediately clean all the joints and afflicted muscle areas body parts before massage with warm water and dry completely with a towel. Apply thin layer of oil as reported above and leave for 10 minutes to soak up. Massage with firm hands. Burn through the sticks and other body parts after the massage. Continue massage till symptoms died forever.

....

CURE NO. 8

Take lamb meat with bones 1 KG. (Without white skin or fat... It's essential) and clean it.

Take green onion 0.5 KG, Gin sing 200 g, Black Cardamom 20 g, Nutmeg 10 g, Garlic 250 g.

Take 1 yellow mango seeds (get out the heavy cover and claim out the kernel) Crush the kernel in pieces and pose in the ingredients.

Now lay the bay window in the oven with 1 l water and put all above ingredients with the lamb meat inside.

Cooked with salt to taste and a little olive oil also at the final level. Bring in lunch and dinner respectively.

This is for one day, but patient responsible can stock all the supply (lamb meat and other parts) in kitchen store from the market for 30 days or on a daily basis...

Take sesame oil 0.5 liter, Olive oil 0.5 liter, Mustard oil 0.5 liter... Mix all oils and place in the pan. Take Golden Flax seed 200 g, Flax Seeds 200 g, Tymol seeds 200 g's........ Puts all in mixed oil and pan on fire. Cut all the factors and then strain the oil. Place the petroleum in the bottle or a stadium. Clean all the marijuana cigarettes and body functions before applying oil and have it absorb for 10 minutes then start massaging vigorously. After hacking through the marijuana cigarettes and body parts with cotton.

....

CURE NO. 9

Take lamb meat on neck 1 KG.
(Without fat, It's essential) and clean
it.

Take 1 KG capsicum, Dry ginger 200
g, Black Cardamom 20 g, Nutmeg 20
g, Garlic 250 g. Black seed 100 g.
Take 1 yellow mango stone (remove
the hard cover and take out the kernel)
Crush the kernel in pieces and put in
the ingredients.

Now lay the bay window in the oven
with 1 l water and put all above
ingredients with the lamb meat inside.
Cooked with salt to taste and add a
small olive oil also at the final stage.
Bring in lunch and dinner with brown
bread or brown rice respectively.

This is for one day, but patient
responsible can stock all the supply
(lamb meat and other voices) in
kitchen store from the market for 30
days or on a daily basis........

Take out 3 piece of Okra (lady finger). Trim the top and bottom of Okra and incise slightly in the center (Be careful not to take off the seminal fluids)

Need a bowl of almost glass size, built of clay (without color, Better) put fresh water in the evening. Put three pieces of Okra with one teaspoonful of Tymol seeds and leave below the sky. In the morning, take out Okra and drink this water one hour after your daily breakfast. Cause sure, Tymol seeds should not be broken up anymore and leave them settled in a layer on the underside of the trough.

Pick out your breakfast with brown bread + Acacia Honey + Black coffee or as you needed, but not more than one fried egg.

Take 750 g, sesame oil and750 g, olive oil........ Mix both oils, then set in the pan. Take 40 shafts of capsicum with seeds (take out with a knife from whole capsicum), 40 shafts of garlic (take out all the garlic bulbs separately for daily use and occupy the center long shaft from bottom bushy parts to clean), Tymol seeds 250 g, Nutmeg 250 g, Mace 250 g's... Crush all as possible and put all in mix oil and pan on fire. Burn all the ingredients and then filter the oil. Put the oil in the bottle or a stadium. Clean all the cannabis cigarettes and body parts before applying oil and have it absorb for 10 minutes then start massaging vigorously. After hacking through the marijuana cigarettes and body parts with cotton.

....

CURE NO. 10

Take 1 KG Toasted white chick peas, 1 KG Toasted black chick peas. 2 KG long black Dates, 1 KG Royal Jelly, 1 KG Olive oil, 0.5 KG Rose Petals. 20 g, Musk...

Take 1 KG whole wheat (crushed) and toast it. Mix white and black chick peas together with toasted crushed wheat. Get out the seed from all the dates... Mix all the ingredients in a large pan. Produce a uniform layer and cut into pieces of 20 g, of candy or biscuit and eat daily one candy after breakfast and one candy noon time with pure rose water.

This is for complete one month usage. Hopefully symptoms of joints pain and muscles afflictions will die completely....

Take 1 KG lamb meat from the neck (without fat, It's essential).... Puts garlic 200 g, ginger 200 g and black pepper 100 g.

Clean the meat and put in the pot full with water, add all the ingredients also in the pot and put on fire. Cook as you like and eat with brown bread and brown rice at lunch and dinner.

This is for one day, but patient responsible can stock all the supply (lamb meat and other ingredients) in kitchen store from the market for 30 days or on a daily basis........

Bring 0.50 liter sesame oil, 0.25 liter mustard oil, 0.50 olive oil, 0.25 walnut oil and mix all oils vigorously than put in the pan.

Take Cloves 200 g, Nutmeg 200 g, Musk 10 g, Mace 200 g... Crush all as possible   except musk. Put all crushed ingredients (except Musk) in mix oil and pan on fire. Incinerate all the ingredients and then sift the oil. Mix Musk in the oil and dissolve it. Then keep the oil in the bottle or a bowl. Clean all the cannabis cigarettes and body parts before applying oil and let it absorb 10 minutes. Afterwards, in the massage vigorously and spread over the joints, body parts with cotton.

....

END

www.ingramcontent.com/pod-product-compliance
Lightning Source LLC
Chambersburg PA
CBHW030551290526
45786CB00004B/1967